THE RECOVERY PLAYBOOK
By Coach Stan Norgalis

How to recover your body between workouts and be prepared for your next training session.

PREFACE AND HOW TO USE THIS BOOK

Many athletes over-train and under-recover. The inspiration for this book is born out of my many years of experience in training and coaching CrossFit, my tenure as a high school basketball coach in New York City, and all of the athletes that I have had (and still have) the pleasure to coach and work with along the way. Your dedication to doing difficult things inspires me and it is the joy of my life to be a part of. This book has been written for you. The goal of this book is to help your body feel consistently strong and vibrant during training session after training session by focusing on what you do *in between* workouts. I hope to inspire you to take your recovery seriously.

At the age of 54, I love to train. 2+ hours a day, 6 days a week, and sometimes multiple sessions in a day. In order to do this, I need my body to be at its best so that I can feel strong, enjoy my training, and most importantly, avoid injury. There are many of us, especially in CrossFit, boot camps, Spartan Races, whatever, who love what we do. *We can't do it if we are injured.*

Here is the playbook that has been effective for me in getting recovered and training hard daily. It has been developed over time and I would encourage you to use it by paying attention to the feedback that your body gives you in training. Take the information, do your own research, consult with your own healthcare provider, and use it to design *your own personal recovery protocol.*

I am confident that if used in this way, the book will be a great partner to you in getting recovered, avoiding injury, and achieving your goals.

DISCLAIMER

The information in this book is for informational and educational purposes only. It is not a substitute for professional medical advice. Accordingly, before taking any action based upon the information in this book, you are encouraged to consult with the appropriate physician or medical professional. The use of any information contained in this book is solely and exclusively at your own risk.

'What you get by achieving your goals isn't as important as what you become by achieving your goals' -Coach Stan

TABLE OF CONTENTS

1. **WATER**....................................page 6
2. **PROTEIN**...............................page 8
3. **BODYWORK**.........................…..page 15
4. **NUTRITION & SUPPLEMENTS**……page 31
5. **PUTTING IT TOGETHER**………………page 44

CHAPTER 1: WATER

Everybody knows the importance of water to the human body. Our bodies are made up of mostly water, and many people are interested to learn that water makes up about 60% of our total body weight. Our particular focus here, as consistent with the title of this book, will be the function of water as it pertains to recovering the body from a training session and preparing it for the next one.

From a recovery perspective, water has 2 main jobs. 1. Hydration of the cells and 2. Cleansing the body of toxins, and in particular, lactic acid.

1. HYDRATION

Quick story. Before class one day, some of the athletes were having a discussion about drinking more water. One of them said "I know that I should drink more water, but when I do, I am always peeing!". In other words, water was not being retained by the body for cellular use. It was bypassing cells and going from the stomach almost directly to the kidneys for removal from the body. This is great for cleansing the bowels but not great for hydrating the body during or outside of a workout.

ENTER THE ALMIGHTY ELECTROLYTE

Think about a wealthy, upscale, country club. The kind where you cannot get in unless you are a member. But wait. Is there a way for you to get in if you are not a member? Yes. Most country clubs have a 'guest policy' where you can get in at any time and enjoy all of the amenities of the club if you are entering with a member who brings you in!

In order for water to enter the cells of your body that perform various functions, electrolytes MUST be present. Electrolytes are the members of the cellular club that allow for water to transport into the cell. The cell is the country club, water is a (most desired) guest, and electrolytes are the members of the club that make it happen.

Water cannot get into the cells without electrolytes. The human body can live for a long time without food. The human body CANNOT live for a long time without electrolytes. Electrolytes are crucial to all bodily processes. Here are the 5 main electrolytes listed below:

SODIUM
POTASSIUM
CHLORIDE
MAGNESIUM
CALCIUM

I cannot emphasize enough the importance of electrolytes, in particular sodium and potassium, to the training athlete or humans in any undertaking that demands high energy production sustained day after day. Many top performers will supplement with electrolyte drinks even before their first cup of coffee!

Recovery and preparation for your next workout, training session, or physical activity begins IMMEDIATELY following your current training session. Priority number one must be replenishing electrolytes. Muscles and energy systems simply cannot function properly without them. With regard to recovery, hydration and the rehydration of cells is how you avoid fatigue, cramping, and put yourself in a position to enjoy your training time.

2. CLEANSING

Water dilutes things. Water rinses things. Water cleans things. In other words, dilute it, rinse it, and now it's clean. Just like doing the dishes ha! The removal of lactic acid is very important to restore optimum function of the muscle cells and have you feeling fresh for your next training session. The oxygen and hydrogen in a water molecule do just that. They bind to the lactic acid and dilute it thus making it easier to leave the muscle.

It is important to note that the rate at which lactate will leave the muscle (and body) can be increased. The lymphatic system, which transports toxins out of the body, does not have a pump. It requires blood flow and movement to transport toxins.

As you hydrate post workout, movement activities like foam rolling, massage, walking, yoga etc. will encourage the lymph to remove ALL of the toxins in your body faster, not just lactate!

Finally, it is paramount to know that lactate can also be used for fuel. Recycled, if you will. Humans all have 2 types of muscle fibers- 1. Fast twitch and 2. Slow twitch.

Here is where the study of the human body gets super cool.

The lactate that is produced by the fast twitch muscle fibers during high intensity training can be USED by the slow twitch muscle fibers for fuel. So those lower intensity activities (like walking) and helping to clear lactate by actually feeding on it.

Now optimizing recovery from a hydrating and cleansing perspective becomes clear. Follow the trifecta of water, massage* , and movement to clear lactate and allow the muscles to spend more time repairing and growing!

*massage being defined as anything that manipulates the muscles out of its resting state like foam rolling, yoga, or actual hand massage.

Hopefully you now have some clarity around water, hydration and the importance of electrolytes to support training and recovery. Let's move on to PROTEIN.

CHAPTER 2 PROTEIN:

pro·tein

[ˈprōˌtēn]
NOUN

1. any of a class of nitrogenous organic compounds that have large molecules composed of one or more long chains of amino acids and are an essential part of all living organisms, especially as structural components of body tissues such as muscle, hair, etc., and as enzymes and antibodies:
   "a protein found in wheat" · "animal proteins"
2. food consisting largely of proteins and making up one of the main nutritional food groups:
   "a diet high in protein" · "Colorado lamb is world-renowned and an excellent source of protein and key nutrients" · "research finds that most people eat proteins fairly unevenly throughout the day"

Simply put, protein is hardware. Think Home Depot. You go to Home Depot to buy the hardware needed to build stuff or repair stuff. Muscles are made of protein and the building blocks of that muscle, if you break it down into its parts, are called amino acids.

Training puts demands on the muscles, which become fatigued and also incur microscopic tears during exercise. An abundance of these tears, especially during the initial phase of an exercise program, results in soreness that may take a while to get rid of as the muscles repair and adapt. In addition, someone who is well conditioned may still feel soreness when new personal records are hit or after training sessions that are especially grueling. Lastly, it is important to note that the connective tissue of bones, tendons, and ligaments (yes, made of protein!) are also stressed during training and need to recover.

If given time, all of the above will heal in due course but what if your goal, like many who do CrossFit or some other type of training that they love, is to recover the body in a day (or less) and be able to safely and effectively hit their next session? Or hit consecutive sessions on consecutive days? Or train everyday?

Full disclosure, I am 54 years old and a six days a week, 2-3 hours a day guy. I love to train and CrossFit is my drug of choice. I train as a professional athlete and in addition, gather all the benefits that being dedicated to a higher purpose brings to an individual.

It also helps me learn a lot on how to recover my body so that I can coach, teach, and help others from the viewpoint of experience.

Fun fact about the human body, it is constantly recycling broken down, dysfunctional proteins. Especially when fasting or practicing time restricted eating. But more on that in my next book haha it is just something folks should be aware of, back to recovery!...

When you train consistently, let's say 4-6 days a week, (e.g.CrossFit, Spartan race training, Strongman, HIIT, etc..), the body requires more exogenous (from the outside) protein to recover and prepare itself for the next training session ON TIME.

How much protein and what types of protein we will get to shortly, but for now you should understand that the body will 1. take proteins you eat 2. Break them down into amino acids and 3. Use those amino acids to build and repair muscle, ligaments, tendons, bones, etc..

Another important item to understand is that there are 9 essential amino acids that allow the human body to function properly and *that it cannot produce on its own. These must be obtained from exogenous sources. Foods that provide all 9 essential amino acids are usually referred to as complete proteins.* Do not confuse non-essential amino acids as 'less important'. Quite the contrary, they are important but the body is able to produce them on its own.

TYPES OF PROTEIN

As we touched on before, let us first understand that there are 21 amino acids that the human body requires for optimum performance. 12 of which the body can produce on its own and 9 of which it cannot. The 9 types of aminos that cannot be produced are called **essential amino acids.** Any food that contains all 9 of these essential aminos is referred to as a **complete protein.**

With regards to recovering quickly and preparing the body for the next day of training many athletes choose to focus on eating complete proteins. One reason is that it simply leaves them less overall eating to do! It is important to note that foods with incomplete proteins (let's say black beans and wheat, as an example) can be combined to make a complete protein.

Complete Proteins: Foods that contain all 9 essential amino acids and have good 'amino density'.

Fish
Poultry
Eggs
Beef
Pork
Dairy
Soy

Also complete proteins but are less amino dense.

Quinoa
Buckwheat
Hemp
Chia

Incomplete proteins: Foods that contain good amounts of protein but lack all of the essential 9 amino acids.

All other Legumes, Nuts, Seeds, and Grains not mentioned above. As an example, black beans have almost as much protein as beef but do not contain all 9 essential amino acids.

So now you can see that for recovery purposes, the athlete has something to think about. It isn't so easy to just throw out a number of 'grams of protein per bodyweight' as a guide of how much protein to eat. 100 grams of chicken protein, as an example, is different in amino *content* than 100 grams of legume or seed protein. So……

HOW MUCH PROTEIN IS NEEDED TO RECOVER THE BODY?

Let me be crystal clear on this one: this is your canvas to paint. You need to put in the thought, time, and be willing to experiment with yourself. And then pay attention to feedback that your body gives you during training.

As an example, I did a nutrition challenge once and was told to eat my bodyweight (190lbs) in grams of protein, which seems to be a popular rule of thumb. Sorry to those well-meaning coaches but that never happened. To this day I can count on one hand the amount of times that I have eaten my bodyweight in protein. However, I can also say that just about *everyday* my body feels fully recovered, and ready for CrossFit activities, in 24 hours or less. (And remember, I am 54 years old).

Today's training (my sixth consecutive day) consisted of 2 strength sessions- clean & jerks and deadlifts followed by a 40 minute EMOM (that's 40 rounds of exercise executed every minute on the minute- thank you HWPO programming). I felt strong and energetic. As I am writing this I decided to add up the grams of protein that I ate yesterday and provide you the types:

60 grams of various plant protein
65 grams of animal protein
20 grams of collagen protein
15 grams of casein protein

This works out to 160 grams of protein. Since my eating doesn't really vary much from day to day, I am probably around this number daily with maybe a 15 gram swing either way.

Again, you need to do you. I would definitely recommend erring on the side of eating too much protein to support high intensity training. But the critical point here is *how does your body feel the next day? When it is your 3rd, 4th, or 5th day in a row and your muscles feel recovered, strong and ready to work,* you know that you found the right protein formula.

Hopefully that provided you with some understanding and guidance around protein and recovery. The goal here is for you to use this information and the chapters that follow *to develop your own, sustainable, recovery protocol.*

CHAPTER 3: MOVEMENT AND BODYWORK

Movement is medicine.

Repeat that. Write it down. Memorize it.

The human body is incredible, amazing, and *highly intuitive*. Its ability to receive stimulus, adapt accordingly, and regenerate itself is truly the first, second, and third wonders of the world.

In order to have a meaningful discussion on using movement and bodywork to recover from training, we must first understand some basic anatomy.

BONES: Levers that move the body in space. Made of mostly collagen protein.

MUSCLES: Organs that act on bones and make them move. Made up of several different proteins including some collagen.

TENDONS: Fibrous tissue that connects muscles to bones. Made up primarily of collagen protein.

LIGAMENTS: Fibrous tissue that connects bone to bone. Made up primarily of collagen protein.

FASCIA: A 'spider web' of connective tissue that holds all of the muscles, organs, nerves, and blood vessels in place. Has a significant amount of sensory nerve endings. Primarily made up of collagen protein.

Two more terms that must be understood, especially with regard to how they differ from each other, are *flexibility and pliability.*

FLEXIBILITY: The range of motion of a joint or sequence of joints.

PLIABILITY: The ability of the muscle to move freely and easily within the fascia (web) that surrounds it.

FLEXIBILITY - (The range of motion of a joint)

For someone on a training, fitness, or workout journey it is important to always work on flexibility. This involves gently stretching muscles, (and therefore) tendons, until they become lengthened over time and new ranges of motion are achieved. Think yoga. And yes, good flexibility helps prevent injury and you will be able to execute training movements with proper technique. Take a back squat or a snatch as an example, it is crucial to perform these movements with proper technique. Your range of motion either allows or disallows for this. Quality of movement trumps everything else with regard to physical training, therefore it is vital for you to work on your flexibility.

Unlike yoga practitioners, you do not need to spend hours and hours in order to move better and improve flexibility. 8 to 15 minutes a day/night, *done consistently,* will provide tremendous benefits with minimal time invested. My personal rule of thumb is to do 15 minutes of stretching every night with 8 minutes being a minimum work requirement. I usually use my mobility app, GO WOD, which takes the thinking out of the process. I just fire up the app and do what I'm told for 15 minutes. This also sends a signal to the body that it is time to relax for bed and I believe this promotes better sleep.

Success Principle: If you are strategic and *consistent* you will be amazed with what you can accomplish over time. Whether the topic is flexibility or something else. Quality over quantity. "It's hard by the yard but a cinch by the inch".

PLIABILITY - (How easily the muscles moves within the fascia)

Do you want to work toward training or fitness goals and achieve them?

Do you want to hit that personal record, make the team, execute that movement you didn't think you could?

Do you want to significantly lower your probability of getting injured while training?

Stop right here and pause for a second.

Now continue.

In my experience, the pliability of your muscles is the top factor in getting recovered, preventing injury, and being able to physically train with consistency. The reason lies in point number two of the last sentence. If you get injured, you cannot train. As you develop your own personal recovery program, muscle pliability must be given a top priority. This is commonly referred to as *bodywork.*

Ever get a massage and the masseuse finds a 'knot' in your muscle that is painful for them to rub out? This 'knot' is called a *trigger point.*

KEY CONCEPT: Trigger points are little bundles of muscle fiber that stay taut, or contracted- not pliable. When not properly attended to through bodywork they present a hazard that can lead to problems elsewhere like tendons and ligaments. Not to mention your muscles will not function at their best during training.

Having unattended trigger points negatively affects the pliability of a muscle. Even just a small number of trigger points can increase your risk of pain and injury, inhibit muscle efficiency, and prevent the fascia from its happy free flowing state.

Since the presence of trigger points also affects fascial integrity and pliability, the term *myofascial release* (broad term) can also be applied to many of the same methods used to fix the specific problem of trigger points.

Therefore, attending to trigger points must be given top priority in any good recovery program

Methods to alleviate trigger points and release restrictions to the fascia:

1. **Foam Rolling:** In terms of time spent, money spent, and degree of effectiveness- foam rolling is in a class by itself. For the

various things that you can do to treat trigger points, release fascia, and keep muscles pliable, foam rolling really has no peer.

The foam roller is a massage tool shaped like a cylinder. The cylinder itself is made of hard plastic and it is surrounded by a layer of foam cushion. Other variations are made of solid styrofoam and others are even electric and create a vibration while being used. All are effective!

There are hundreds of videos on the internet on how to use foam rollers. What it is important for you to understand is that foam rolling is a great way to:

A. Massage, lengthen, and increase blood flow around the muscles.
B. Become aware of trigger points and *roll them out* anytime in between training sessions (and even during!).
C. Prepare muscles to be exercised and begin recovering them after exercise.

Foam rolling does not take a lot of time to get the job done. As an example, **pre-workout** you can spend 20 to 30 seconds on every major body part and have done a thorough job in 6-8 minutes. The muscles and fascia will be left significantly more pliable and ready to work.

Recovery benefits of foam rolling ***post-workout*** include its ability to move lactic acid out of the muscles. **Enhancing lactate clearance is of utmost importance in recovery and preparing for your next training session.**

Smart athletes begin recovering for their next training session immediately after the current one is over.

Benefits of post workout foam rolling:

A. It is an important way to facilitate lactate clearance.

B. Smooths out muscles and fascia preventing trigger points and treating ones that have been created during exercise.

C. It is a great way to freshen up the muscles *during* training sessions when you have a break or are doing interval training.

All of the above are great at preventing injuries, will leave muscles less sore in between sessions, and will leave the body feeling more limber and loose for all training activities. For me personally, I do not begin a training session until I have rolled out.

The final benefit that I will mention is cost. The only monetary investment you will make is purchasing the foam roller itself. The cost is quite inexpensive compared to the quantity of use that you get out of them (a good one lasts a very long time). A good quality foam roller will run you $20 to $40 with the vibrating ones being more expensive than that.

Combining cost with all of the benefits mentioned prior, and you can understand why I recommend foam rolling as *the* integral part of your personal recovery program.

2. **Massage Balls:** While foam rolling is your global workhorse for muscle pliability, myofascial, and trigger point release: a good massage ball is a great compliment to that protocol.

Massage balls are made of hard rubber and vary in size between that of a lacrosse ball (which I actually use for massaging my feet by simply standing on it then moving it around) and that of a softball. The surface is usually contoured so that it can grasp onto parts of the skin and not slip away.

Trigger points can be stubborn and require some 'tough love'. The massage ball provides a way to target a specific 'knot' and break it up by applying direct pressure into the same point repeatedly. This specific pressure, also known as *'mashing'*, can be quite painful and yet very effective in reducing or eliminating trigger points.

This is similar to the Japanese style of massage, called shiatsu, where the masseuse will use their fingers to painfully manipulate muscle knots and release fascia. The massage ball provides a way for you to do this style of massage to yourself.

Keep in mind that foam rolling is also feedback. If there is a spot on your body that is particularly painful while rolling, you have a good indicator that a more targeted release is needed on that spot. You may want to 'go after' that spot later with a massage ball or the foam roller.

My personal recovery protocol involves 15-20 minutes of yoga every night. I will also use this time to use my massage ball and target specific areas depending on the feedback I received while foam rolling earlier in the day.

NOTE: The human body is *very* intuitive. It receives signals and then adapts and acts accordingly. Building in 15 or so minutes of yoga and gentle stretching before bed sends a signal to your body that it is time to *relax.* Muscles are being given a message that they have some time off! You will sleep better and some of those milder trigger points may even loosen up and free themselves while you're sleeping!

3. **Static Stretching and Yoga:** This is your traditional method of flexibility training which involves gently moving muscles and joints out of their 'comfort zone'. The joint(s) is then held for a period of time in a stretched state relative to its resting range of motion. Like foam rolling there and thousands of videos and many apps that can show you different methods of stretching and yoga.

Keep in mind that using stretching to increase range of motion, which is a highly desirable outcome, *takes time.* This is another example of how a little at a time, performed with *consistency,* is what gets the job done. It is far better to stretch for 15 minutes a day than longer periods of time done infrequently.

There is also **ballistic stretching** where the joints and muscles are moved into a stretched state for only a moment, then allowed back to their resting length, and repeated several times. This is usually used by athletes pre-workout to warm up muscles for repeated contraction (activity).

Stretching and yoga have several benefits as part of a well rounded recovery program:

A. They help muscles recover faster post training session by improving circulation, leaving muscles and joints feeling less sore.

B. By elongating the muscle and holding it there, the tendency to create new trigger points can be significantly reduced as the muscle is being given the sensory message to relax.

C. Over time, stretching increases flexibility and mobility resulting in better movement patterns that reduce the risk of all-cause injury. (Read 'C' again!)

As far as my personal protocol, I will do a little bit of stretching all the time. In between warm up exercises, in between sets of training exercises, and as part of my cool down after a workout. At night I use a mobility app and plug in a 15 minute guided yoga session.

As you gain an understanding of your mobility challenges and concerns, you will develop your own protocol of 'go to' stretches that keep you feeling good, out of harm's way, and increase your range of motion.

Think of stretching as dividends paid to you from a healthy company: little by little, a little becomes a lot. Small amounts of stretching done consistently provide many recovery and training benefits. Build them into your daily recovery protocol.

I am a big believer in efficiency. Especially when it comes to behavior change, working toward goals, and time management. I like small tasks with big payoffs. The trifecta of foam rolling, massage balls, and stretching have big payoffs relative to time and money spent. Also, these activities can be done by yourself, you are not dependent on others to help, and they adapt to many different surroundings.

Note: As we get further into things that you can do for bodywork, keep in mind that these three can keep you feeling great and training well day after day. You do not need to add more unless you want to.

4. **Cold Therapy:** Continuing the discussion of powerful recovery protocols that cost little or no money I would be remiss not to mention this powerhouse. Cold therapy can be simply immersing your body in a cold tub or taking a cold shower. Lakes and oceans work well too!

The foundation of cold therapy is the slowing down of inflammatory signals while the body is made cold and then an uptick of anti-inflammatory proteins when normal blood flow returns to the area.

Cold water is a super way to reduce the inflammation that is caused by physical exertion. There are numerous other reported health benefits (reducing stress response, boosting the immune system, improved mood, etc.) to this protocol, it costs nothing, and doesn't take a lot of time. My personal method is to take my normal warm shower post-training, clean myself, and then turn the knob all the way to cold for 5-6 minutes. I do this after every workout.

Another benefit that I have experienced from cold showers and baths, is a big uptick in my own mental toughness. When it's the middle of winter and you are able to withstand bone chilling water hitting your body, your mind becomes quite resilient to many other hardships of life- in and out of the gym.

In addition, cold therapy causes the release of *cold shock proteins* within the body. These proteins can help cells regenerate, support the immune system, and even protect your brain.

Yes, cold therapy does include your traditional ice pack or bag of ice on a particular sore body part- usually for about 10-15 minutes. Also, some folks like to purchase their own special bathtubs (ice cubes and water) for cold immersion or go to centers for *cryotherapy.*

Cryotherapy centers are where people go to a facility and immerse themselves in a tank or booth which is then blasted for 3-5 minutes with ice cold vapor (usually nitrogen). There is a cost for this in both money and time spent getting to the facility. I recommend reading up on cryotherapy to determine if it is right for you.

Lastly, cold water therapy has a stimulating effect on the lymphatic system. This is the system that destroys bacteria and damaged cells. It is a crucial part of keeping us healthy! The contraction and subsequent expansion of blood vessels caused by cold therapy keeps the lymph active and working at a high level.

Before we get into additional bodywork methods should you have the time and money, let's put some thought into using what we have up until this point. It is important for you to understand how small amounts of time spent add up!

Snapshot of potential weekly bodywork:

Pre-workout: 6-8 minutes of foam rolling
Post-workout: 6-8 minutes of foam rolling, massage ball, and/or stretching
Cold shower: 5 minutes
Bedtime (or any other time) Yoga/Stretching: 10-15 minutes

Total time spent taking care of your body: 27-36 minutes

Let's say you follow this protocol 5 days a week: That means you will be spending 135-180 minutes (that's 2-3 hours!) taking care of your body and recovering for your next training session. Small amounts of time add up!

Ok, moving on now…

ACTIVE RECOVERY

If you have the time, active recovery can be a very powerful tool in your recovery protocol. Active recovery can look like a lot of different things but the overriding theme is: *low intensity movement.*

The science behind low intensity activity for recovery is simple. Low intensity work uses slow twitch muscle fibers to do the activity. Some examples are going for a walk, a super slow jog or easily pedaling a stationary bike.

The beauty of slow twitch muscle fibers is that they will use lactic acid (lactate) for fuel. If you have built up substantial lactate during a high intensity training session, leaving muscles tired and sore, the slow movement provides an opportunity for the lactate to get used up. This is also referred to as a lactic acid *flush*. Even just 10-20 minutes of low intensity movement can go a long way in clearing lactate. The more you clear, the fresher you will feel for your next training session.

In addition, be mindful that active recovery is a great way to spend 'off' days from training. Movement is medicine both physically and mentally. Activity and enjoying things in nature like swimming, hiking, biking, etc are all good for the mind, body, and spirit. They are also fantastic for freshening up the body!

3 MORE ALTERNATIVE RECOVERY METHODS DEPENDING ON YOUR TIME AND FINANCIAL ABILITY.

1. **Acupuncture:** By definition, acupuncture is a type of Chinese Medicine. It is performed by setting needles into the outermost layer of skin and leaving them there for a period of time. The premise of acupuncture is that the human body has 'energy channels' called *meridians.*

The practitioner will place needles into the skin with the goal of stimulating the meridians to induce healing. Acupuncture has been known to treat many types of ailments including muscle and joint pain, disease, and stimulate proper organ function. I personally used acupuncture to successfully heal a tear of a rotator cuff muscle in my shoulder.

A good acupuncturist can also use the needles to treat trigger points!

Rather than leave the needles in the skin, the practitioner will set the needle directly into a trigger point, the muscle will spasm releasing the trigger point, and then they will instantaneously remove the needle. This is an incredibly effective way to alleviate muscle knots.

2. **Chiropractic Care:** A chiropractor is a *hands-on* health professional with extensive training in anatomy and kinesiology. They will physically use their hands to treat and rebalance skeletal muscle, joints, and fascia.

For someone leading an active lifestyle, a good chiropractor can be extremely valuable. Regular check-ins can treat skeletal and muscular issues before they become chronic, prevent new problems from arising, and induce myofascial (trigger point) release- which by now you are understanding is a pretty big deal!

I would look for a practitioner who is certified in ART*- Active Release Technique.

*This indicates that they have had specific training in myofascial release.

Both acupuncture and chiropractic care are covered under many insurance plans. There is usually a deductible or a co-pay.

3. **Massage:** A good massage needs no introduction: It is relaxing to the muscles, stimulating to the lymphatic system which removes toxins, and a great way to de-stress. A few types to highlight regarding recovery.

A. Foot reflexology: *"Strength starts from the feet"- Chinese saying.* The feet are largely forgotten about and taken for granted in training yet everything that you do goes through your feet! Foot reflexology is massage that is dedicated to the foot and lower leg by targeting specific points (similar to the meridians in acupuncture) and varying the pressure applied to them. There are thousands of nerves in the feet and when they are stimulated through reflexology, they provide numerous mental and physical health benefits. Plus, it just feels great! The good news is that while not covered by insurance, a session is usually pretty reasonably priced (I pay $30 for 30 minutes.) **IMPORTANT:** Using a massage ball by stepping on it and moving it around your arch and foot is a most beneficial and inexpensive way to give yourself foot reflexology. Keep this in the front of your mind!

B. Shiatsu/Qi Gong/Acupressure: Are all forms of 'stronger' massage types geared toward myofascial and trigger point release. Shiatsu has a reputation for being particularly painful and yet very effective.

C. Swedish: A whole body massage that is more relaxing and calming rather than strong and/or painful. It relieves muscle tension and increases blood flow and lymph activity. A nice reward after a good run of training days!

D. Cupping: While not exactly a massage, I felt like cupping should be included here. Cupping involves 'suction cups' which are vacuum sealed onto the skin and generate intense blood flow to a specific area. Cupping does cause bruising to the skin but not the underlying muscle. The premise of cupping is that when the capillaries are broken down (hence the bruising) and rebuilt, blood flow and healing to that particular area are improved.

E. Scraping: An intense form of massage originating in China, the practitioner will use a blade like metal object, called a *gua sha* on trigger points and fascia, and literally 'scrape' into the tissue. Scraping will burst capillaries in a similar fashion to cupping. This can be quite painful yet also very effective at reducing trigger points and restoring proper muscle function. Scraping alters the angle at which tissue is manipulated. This provides an opportunity for stubborn trigger points to be alleviated and proper fascial integrity to be restored.

F. Electric Stimulation (E-Stim): Sensors are placed on the skin (similar to and EKG machine) and mild electronic pulses send 'shocks' to the treatment area. 'TENS' units (stand for Transcutaneous Electric Nerve Stimulation) are a popular machine used to deliver this type of treatment. It is used for treating trigger points, tendinitis, and any area that may benefit from increased blood flow during recovery. These units are reasonably priced and I have successfully treated tendinitis with mine.

CHAPTER 4: NUTRITION & SUPPLEMENTS

Make sure that you talk to your doctor or healthcare provider regarding changes to your diet or adding supplements. The following information is for educational purposes only.

What I am *not* going to do in this chapter is tell you what and what not to eat. Or what supplements to take or not to take.

What I am going to do for your benefit, is take the subject of what 'we put into our mouth', and provide a way to look at it in the context of recovery and health. As with the prior chapters, this chapter should enable you to build your own nutritional and supplemental protocol that helps you get *consistently* recovered for your next training session.

With regard to recovery (and my health) I view everything that I put into my body into one of three categories, I call it "*The Trifecta of Nutrition*".

1. **Anti Oxidants:** The primary enemy of the human body is *free radical* activity. A 'free radical' is an *oxygen molecule with an unpaired electron.* The electron of an oxygen molecule wants to be paired with another. If no electron is readily available, the free radical will attack healthy cells to find its partner! Antioxidants *provide a donor electron* to the unpaired electron so that it does not attack a healthy cell. Whether you get them through nutrition and/or supplements, it is impossible to overstate the value of antioxidants. Vitamin C is probably the most famous one.

2. **Anti Inflammatory:** Inflammation is how your body understands that something is wrong so that it can attempt to heal itself. Inflammation expresses itself in pain, swelling, bruising, and also disease. It would then follow that we want to ingest things that would reduce pain and inflammation to promote healing between training sessions and throughout life!

3. **Restorative:** The purpose of training is to stress the body so that it must adapt. Restoratives are items that help promote healing and *growth*. As an example, the amino acids that make up protein. For the purposes of this chapter they are food and supplements that *'restore'* muscles, bones, and connective tissue. Restoratives heal and also prepare the body to train again.

Two more terms to understand are *nutrient density* and *energy density*. *Nutrient dense* are foods with a lot of nutrient value (vitamins and minerals) and *energy dense* are foods with a lot of calories that can be used for energy. Calories often get a bad rap but remember that they are simply a way to measure energy. Foods can lean towards being more nutrient dense, more energy dense, or both!

For example:

Say you're going to have some eggs. Good, pasture raised, orange yolk, eggs. (When it comes to eggs, the more orange the yolk, the more nutrients inside.)

As I am checking recovery boxes in my head, I ask myself. What am I getting from the eggs that can help me recover from training? How many of the 3 recovery categories can I check?

Well, amongst the 13 vitamins and minerals in an egg are lutein and zeaxanthin (anti inflammatories), these are also antioxidants, and the peptides in the amino acids are antioxidants. Antioxidants and antiinflammatories, checked.

When we think of restoratives, the egg white is a *complete protein* meaning that it has all 9 essential amino acids for repairing and building tissue. Also restorative, the egg yolk contains the vitamins and minerals plus good fats for *energy* and making hormones. Restoratives, checked.

Because you not only get a lot of nutrients in the egg but a good amount of calories in fat and protein, you can consider the egg both *nutrient dense* and *energy dense*.

Another example of this would be an avocado. Avocados have a high concentration of omega-9 fatty acids which are anti-inflammatory, a good amount of minerals, and also have a solid calorie content. So again you have nutrient density and energy density.

Another way to look at these is through the terms *micronutrients* (micros) and *macronutrients* (macros). Micronutrients being your vitamins and minerals. Macronutrients being your protein, fat, and carbohydrate. Eggs and avocados, as an example, have a good amount of both macro and micro nutrients.

On the other end of the spectrum take spinach. Very high in vitamins and minerals but not a lot of calories. Nutrient dense? Yes. Energy dense? No. How about a burger, fries and soda from your favorite fast food chain? Energy dense? Hell, yes. Lots of calories. Nutrient dense? No. Significantly lacking in vitamins and minerals.

There is an old saying "you can't out train a shitty diet". Keep that in mind when making choices that affect your recovery. I enjoy some 'fun food' once in a while (my go to is coffee or pistachio ice cream) and by all means crush that pizza when you need to, but for the most part think: antioxidants, anti-inflammatories, and nutrient dense macros for restoring the body between workouts.

A NOTE ON FATTY ACIDS & INFLAMMATION

I will now provide another example of how the quality of the food you eat matters. There are 3 types of fatty acids in food: omega-3, omega-6, and omega-9. These are important because the overall ratio of them inside your body either contribute to or reduce the inflammatory response. Your ratio of omega 6 to omega 3 & 9 is not only significant for recovery but also *your overall health.*

Omega 3 and omega 9 are *anti-inflammatory* fatty acids while omega 6 is *pro-inflammatory.* Remember, we want to ingest anti-inflammatory foods and supplements because reducing inflammation will help our recovery process (this also helps the body against disease and illness). By now you've got it, more omega 3 and 9, less omega 6.

How do we look at food through this lens of fatty acids?

Let's use grass fed beef as our example. The term 'grass fed' refers to the cattle being allowed to graze and feed off the land at their leisure. Grass fed beef has a high concentration of omega 3 fatty acids (and also an extensive micronutrient profile). However, that same beef, when it is mass produced and the cattle are given a poor diet with added hormones (to make it grow faster) - *now produces a beef dominant in omega 6 fats and far less micronutrients.* The way in which animals are fed and raised has a huge effect on the nutrient density of the food you eat! On a side note, wild caught fish or a high quality fish oil supplement are great ways to increase the omega 3 in your diet.

Key terms to help you shop for food:

When it comes to meats, fruits, and vegetables we are looking for the terms *organic, grass fed, pasture raised, wild caught, and of course non-gmo* (meaning genetically modified organisms were not used in the production of the food). Both the macronutrient and micronutrient profile of these foods will be **much** higher and therefore better for recovering the body and your overall health.

Regardless of what eating style you follow: Meat & Vegetables, Vegan, Keto, Paleo, Time restricted eating (intermittent fasting), 3 meals a day, small meals throughout the day or a little bit of everything..

Measure using *The Trifecta:*

1. Am I getting antioxidants to combat free radical damage?
2. Am I eating anti-inflammatory or pro-inflammatory foods?
3. Am I eating foods that will restore me by healing body tissue and providing fuel for my next training session?

If you are checking 1, 2, or all 3 of these on a particular food item then you are on the right track. Looking up items on the internet becomes super helpful as you design and create your own personal eating style. Simple ways to ask the internet questions:

"Is grass fed beef anti inflammatory"
"Does olive oil have omega 3 fatty acids?"
"Are eggs a complete protein?"
"What are foods that contain omega 6 fatty acids?"
"Are avocados high in antioxidants?"

Research for the win. Use the internet and find out about your foods- we all know that you're staring at your phone anyway!

A little bit of research combined with the principles outlined above and you will quickly be a pro at understanding nutrient profiles. This not only helps you recover from and for training but be healthier overall!

SUPPLEMENTS

Supplements can be helpful because they can *supplement* the foods you eat in recovering the body and preparing for your next training session. Also, depending on activity levels, nutrition and sleep, supplements may be more or less needed. Some other ways that supplements can be helpful:

A. They target deficiencies in needed recovery nutrients.

B. When tracking calories for weight management they can help get nutrients into the body with little or no caloric value.

C. They are a time saver in the context of a busy lifestyle, especially when you can't eat properly.

Please keep in mind that this book is largely (but not exclusively) written for athletes who are training consecutive days in a row. Let's call it 4-6 days a week. I witness this all the time at the CrossFit gyms that I coach in where it is common for people to come 5 or 6 days of the week and train at high intensity. This would extend to athletes competing in sport, Spartan Races, etc..

Someone who is working out for an hour, 3 days a week, may or may not need supplements as they can get everything that they need for recovery from their day to day nutrition combined with the other items in this book.

Where to start

First and foremost, restorative supplements are a priority. They will help repair muscle and connective tissue, assist in the growth of muscle and connective tissue, and store fuel to be used in the next training period. Important work! Let's break down some of these.

Protein and amino acids

Logically, a big part of this discussion would be about protein and amino acids. The most popular supplements being protein shakes (of which there are many that you can buy pre-made or you can make your own) and also amino acid powders, drinks, and capsules.

Protein shakes will usually come with some calories to consider (that may be much needed to store fuel) whereas amino acids supplements will not. The protein has already been broken down for you.

The way that I typically use these variations is amino acids before a workout for fuel (because I want to have an empty stomach before training) and then a home made protein shake(s) after training and or later in the day. I prefer to make my own shakes where I can directly control the ingredients, nutrient density, plus get some antioxidants and anti inflammatories. Here is one of my 'go to' post workout shakes:

1 scoop egg white protein powder 19g protein (restorative)
1 scoop plant protein powder 21g protein (restorative)
1 scoop collagen peptides 10g (restorative)
2 tablespoons of cocoa powder (or cinnamon powder) (antioxidant)
2 tablespoons ground flaxseed or 1 tablespoon mct oil (anti inflammatory)
¼ teaspoon salt (electrolyte)
¼ teaspoon potassium (electrolyte)
5 drops of liquid monk fruit (zero calorie non gmo sweetener)
5mg creatine (restorative, antioxidant)

SIMPLICITY: All of the above ingredients store at room temperature, and are quite easy to keep around in bulk so you always have the ingredients on hand. Note: Cream of tartar in the spice section of the supermarket as is pure potassium.

Just throw them all in a blender with water and ice. It takes me 3-5 minutes to make this shake.

Regarding amino acids, I take glutamine by capsule (glutamine is also a big fuel for the immune system, so 2 benefits for 1 supplement), and drink a mixture of electrolytes and amino acids before I train. This keeps my stomach empty but my body charged up and ready to work.

There are many different ways that people supplement protein shakes and amino acids. I gave you my examples as food for thought. Play around with what works best for you. Remember, you're putting together YOUR recovery program. Play around with different things and if you're feeling *consistently* fresh and ready to train, you have found your formula!

Two other proteins worth mentioning, which I take daily, are collagen and casein (milk protein).

Collagen I take to support my tendons, ligaments, and bone (I mean, collagen is what they are actually made of!) and I consider it a crucial component of my recovery protocol. Bone broth soups or powder form put into shakes or coffee are two ways to add collagen. The more 'natural' you can take collagen or any supplement in, the better.

Casein protein, found in cow's milk, contains all nine essential amino acids. Considered a 'slow release' protein because it is digested slower, casein allows for more protein to be utilized for repair and growth. The last thing that I eat on any given day is a skyr or greek yogurt for its casein value.

Both of these proteins are super-restorative in my opinion and I recommend taking them post-training session. Keep in mind that your body does its healing, repairing, and *growing* at night while you sleep!

Regardless of how you go about using protein and amino acids, as always, I would recommend 'clean' ingredients. Non GMO, labels that you can understand what's in it, and of course organic if possible.

Creatine

You probably saw creatine as an additive to my shake. It is one of the most widely studied supplements of all time. Far too many pre and post workout benefits to itemize here. Some studies even suggest it helps people live longer. Don't take my word, read up on it!

Vitamin C, Turmeric, Zinc

Most people understand Vitamin C as helping your immune system prevent or shorten the duration of colds. And yes, it is a powerful antioxidant. And yes, training does spike the activity of free radicals so an antioxidant supplement like vitamin C makes sense.

What many people do not know about vitamin C is that it is a key nutrient in the formation of bones and connective tissue. As an example, it is a direct partner to your collagen supplement. Vitamin C is needed to form new blood vessels and even helps in the production of anabolic hormones like testosterone. So Vitamin C is also restorative.

Rounding out the trifecta, vitamin C also has anti-inflammatory properties, making it a great all around supplement to support recovery for training. I keep vitamin C with me all the time and will take small doses throughout the day while I am coaching. If you are just going to take it once a day I would recommend before bed since that is when the majority of healing will take place.

Zinc and Turmeric are 2 other noteworthy supplements. Turmeric is widely known for being a strong antioxidant and anti-inflammatory. Zinc is not only a great antioxidant but also helps muscles repair and grow (restorative). I take both of these daily. Another great aspect of Vitamin C, Zinc and turmeric is that they are quite inexpensive relative to the world of supplements. You can really upgrade your recovery and overall health at a minimal expense.

B Complex Vitamins:

B Vitamins are responsible for metabolizing the foods that you eat into energy. I take a B Complex vitamin pre-training session.

Recovery drinks

Post-workout, I drink a *very* low calorie, all natural, recovery drink consisting of amino acids, electrolytes, and vitamins. These are simply the things that I need to get into my body to begin recovery. The reason for the low calories is that I do not want to spike insulin. Rather, I want the full metabolic and longevity benefits occurring from the hormones produced by training. To maximize this, I personally do not eat post training sessions until my body starts asking me for food.

We will stop here as there is literally no end to the discussion on supplements. What I have provided here is some examples of how I do things and why I am doing them. Keep in mind I train 6 days a week for 2+ hours a day.

Play around with what works for you and remember to pay attention to the feedback that your body gives you in the next workout.

Sleep and Sleep Supplements

Needless to say, sleep is an important part of recovery. It is when healing and growth take place. The best sleep supplement is a *routine* also called *sleep hygiene* that cues your body for sleep.

As an example my routine is a shower, followed by 15 minutes of yoga/bodywork, prayer, and then I will like to watch weightlifting videos from around the world with the sound off as this is very relaxing to me. Then I shut the TV off at about the same time every night and sleep.

Going to bed at the same time and sleeping the same hours can be very beneficial if you can pull it off. Our body regulates many systems off of something called circadian rhythms. In simple terms this means sleeping, waking, and eating at the same times everyday.

Now we all know that we live in an imperfect world with imperfect lives so whatever you do, do not worry about your sleep hygiene. Simply work at it like everything else and do the best that you can!

I do take 2 sleep supplements that I have found beneficial. I take 1mg of melatonin (antioxidant) and 500mg of Tryptophan (restorative-the amino acid found in turkey protein that makes everybody sleepy at Thanksgiving).

Through trial and error I have found this combination helps me get a great night's sleep and I am ready to go the next morning.

If you consider a sleep supplement, do your research, and like everything else in this book, speak to your doctor as you try to find what works best for you.

In closing, these are some supplements that work for me and keep me recovered and training well. When considering supplements, be strategic. You do not need every supplement in the world, just keep looking at things as either restorative, antioxidants, or anti inflammation. Pay attention to how you feel physically and mentally in the next training session.

CHAPTER 5:

FINAL THOUGHTS AND PUTTING IT ALL TOGETHER

'Great things can be accomplished if you are willing to be imperfect'-Coach Stan

As a coach, it is my primary job *to take care of people*. To direct their motivations toward their own maximum benefit. There is a lot of simple, functional, and important information in this book. I want athletes to care about their recovery, *especially* the hard working people of all ages who show up at their CrossFit affiliates everyday and get after it. I coach these people and they are my heroes. The dedication that I witness daily was the inspiration for The Recovery Playbook. This book is my way of taking care of as many people as I can.

Unfortunately many people overtrain and under-recover. This leads to fatigue, injuries, and extended time either away from the gym or folks that are limited in what they can do. Not fun. I want you to feel strong, powerful, and ready for action day after day.

The solution is to put together your own living, breathing recovery protocol. It doesn't have to be perfect right away. It doesn't have to take a lot of time. It doesn't have to involve every single item mentioned in this book!

Take the principles and information here and let it evolve. Something is better than nothing.

Here are some guidelines and remember, something is better than nothing!

-Make time for bodywork: pre and post exercise and before bed.

Don't have time for the whole body? Roll the major muscle groups that will be worked today in training. Only have a few minutes after class? Do a quick roll of what got worked to most (quads? hamstrings?) or hit a full body yoga pose for 90 seconds (a wall candle or forward bend are two good ones).

-10-15 minutes of yoga before bed sends a signal to the muscles that it is time to relax. You will sleep better, heal, and grow better.

-Ask your coach to slip 3-4 minutes of stretching into class. I always stretch my athletes after their warmup.

-Post workout nutrition focused on water, electrolytes, and protein.

-Himalayan sea salt is a great inexpensive source for electrolytes.

-Food quality matters: organic, pasture raised, grass fed, non-GMO…

-Find ways to get slow movement in-post training session, 5 minutes here, 10 minutes there. A 15 minute walk? Super.

-Keep a foam roller and/or massage ball near your TV. Use it for 10 minutes. I mean, you binge watch a show for hours right?

-Treat trigger points. The sooner the better.

-Be mindful that tendons and ligaments take more time to adapt to training than muscle. Take your collagen and back off after hitting personal bests.

-Pay attention and reflect on how your *time* is spent. I promise you that you have more time than you think.

-Listen to your body, back off training if you feel sluggish or tired. By all means get something done but live to fight another day.

-Listen to your body if you're feeling great. Go for the Personal Best! Make a checklist in your head of the things that you did to get ready to train. All of my checklist items are in this book!

-Consistency in recovery is going to lead to consistency in training.

-Consistency in training is going to lead to achieving your goals.

-Change takes time, be patient with yourself and keep going.

Everything that you need for recovery is here.
Everything else is already inside of you.

Now go train hard and make yourself proud.

Coach Stan

Made in United States
North Haven, CT
20 August 2023

40520170R00026